The Permanently Beat PCOS Diet & Exercise Shortcuts: Cookbook, Recipes & Exercise

Now Includes 33 Delicious, Healthy, Low Glycemic Index Recipes [Companion to Bestseller "Permanently Beat PCOS: The Complete Solution"]

Caroline D. Greene

Published by Women's Republic

Atlanta, Georgia USA

All Rights Reserved

No part of this book may be reproduced or transmitted for resale or use by any party other than the individual purchaser who is the sole authorized user of this information. Purchaser is authorized to use any of the information in this publication for his or her own use only. All other reproduction or transmission, or any form or by any means, electronic or mechanical, including photocopying, recording or by any informational storage or retrieval system, is prohibited without express written permission from the author.

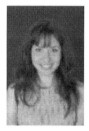

Caroline D. Greene

Copyright © 2012 Caroline D. Greene

What Our Readers Are Saying

"My BMI number is now well within the healthy range and we're going to try for our first child"

★★★★★ Suzie Robertson (Sheffield, AL)

"I just can't believe how simple it was to implement the changes and how tasty they would be!"

★★★★★ Raquel Lampert (Charlton Heights, WV)

"Easy to follow and packed with more than I was expecting - exactly what I needed"

★★★★☆ Justine Patrick (Spurger, TX)

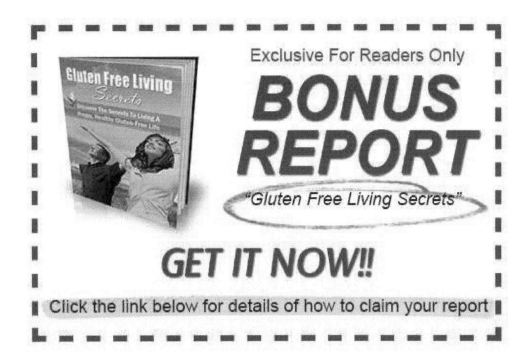

Exclusive Bonus Download: Gluten Free Living Secrets

Are you sick and tired of trying every weight loss program out there and failing to see results? Or are you frustrated with not feeling as energetic as you used to despite what you eat? Perhaps you always seem to have a bit of a " dodgy stomach " and indigestion seems to be a regular part of your life?

There's nothing worse than sitting down to a nice big plate of pasta and enjoying your meal only to be met with a growling stomach and the inevitable rush to the toilet.

It's that bloated feeling you get after eating a piece of bread that just " doesn't seem right " . Almost as if you've eaten something poisonous.

Gluten Free Living Secrets is a complete resource that will tell you everything you need to know about the dangers of eating gluten and how to go about transitioning yourself and your family to a life free of this dangerous substance.

Here's just a taste of what you will discover inside Gluten Free Living Secrets:

- What foods you should focus on when first switching to a gluten-free diet
- The 9 grains that are safe and gluten-free

- The truth about whether you can eat pasta on a gluten-free diet
- What you should know to determine if you have Celiac Disease
- and that's not all...
- Why you may want to consider eliminating gluten from your child's diet
- The top 10 reasons to go gluten-free
- How to transform your pantry to be gluten-free
- A list of essential gluten-free shopping tips
- How to keep your kids happy around their gluten-eating friends
- Tips on staying gluten-free when eating out

Gluten Free Living Secrets comes in a digital PDF format that is easy to read either on your computer or on your eBook reader.

Go to the end of this book for the download link for this Bonus

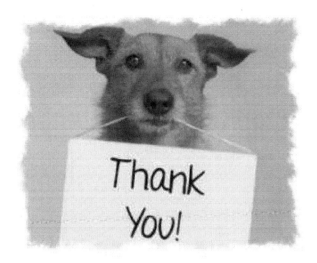

Thank you for downloading my book. Please REVIEW this book on Amazon. I need your feedback to make the next version better. Thank you so much!

Books by This Author

Permanently Beat Bacterial Vaginosis

Permanently Beat Yeast Infection & Candida

Permanently Beat Urinary Tract Infections

Permanently Beat Hypothyroidism Naturally

Permanently Beat PCOS

The Permanently Beat PCOS Diet & Exercise Shortcuts

Author's Foreword

Many thousands of women have already benefitted from having read my first book on the topic of PCOS "*Permanently Beat PCOS: The Complete Solution*", but for those of you who haven't it's important to note that whilst you will benefit by following the advice in this book alone the focus of the two books are quite different. This is book is intended to be a more hands-on, how-to approach for women who already understand their condition and, as such spends far less time on explaining what PCOS is and why it is affecting their health the way it does. By contrast, my first book is aimed at people who need 'the big picture' and goes into detail on what PCOS is and isn't and a much more holistic treatment approach and as such is a great starting point for anyone.

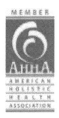

Table of Contents

How to Manage PCOS with Diet and Exercise 11
    Ready…Set…Go! Planning to Exercise Wisely 12
    Building Your Endurance Step by Step, Rep by Rep 13
To burn fat 14
    To Lose or Maintain…That is the Question 14
    Starter Exercise Regiment 15
    Keep It Fresh 'n Fun 25
More Effective Fat-Burning: Your Target Heart Rate 27
Raise Your Metabolic Rate 29
    Eat Smart, Live Well 30
Low Glycemic Diet for PCOS 33
    Lean Meats and Low-Fat Dairy Treats 34
What's On the Menu: Recipes for Women with PCOS 37
    Smoothies 39
    1. Banana and Strawberry Smoothie 39
    2. Vegetable Smoothie 40
    Snacks 41
    3. Potato Crisps 41
    4. Apricot Cookies 42
    5. Herbs Crackers 43
    Breakfast 44
    6. Pancakes made with coconut flour 44
    7. Low-fat Yoghurt with fruit 45
    8. Oats Porridge 46
    9. Fruit and Muesli bread 47
    10. Sweet corn on the cob 48
    11. Stuffed bun with shallots and meat 49
    12. Baked beans in ham sauce 50
    Lunch 51

13. Black Eyed Beans 51
14. Mung Beans fried 52
15. Chick Peas Hummus dip 54
16. Mushroom and spinach Mix 55
17. Chicken Korma 56
18. Basmati white rice with Green peas 57
19. Kidney Beans 58
Dinner 60
20. Penne with Vegetables 60
21. Chili Beef Noodles 61
22. Cumberland Fish Pie 62
23. Vegetable Burger 63
24. Hamburger 65
25. Beef and ale Casserole 67
26. Tomato and herb chicken 68
Deserts 69
27. Apple Berry Crumble 69
28. Mixed Berry Mousse 70
29. Doughnut 71
30. Low-Fat Vanilla Custard 73
31. Rice Pudding Caramel 74
32. Rice Pudding cinnamon flavored 75
33. Chocolate Butterscotch Muffin 76
Exclusive Bonus Download: Gluten Free Living Secrets 78
One Last Thing 80

Disclaimer

While all attempts have been made to provide effective, verifiable information in this Book, neither the Author nor Publisher assumes any responsibility for errors, inaccuracies, or omissions. Any slights of people or organizations are unintentional.

This Book is not a source of medical information, and it should not be regarded as such. This publication is designed to provide accurate and authoritative information in regard to the subject matter covered. It is sold with the understanding that the publisher is not engaged in rendering a medical service. As with any medical advice, the reader is strongly encouraged to seek professional medical advice before taking action.

How to Manage PCOS with Diet and Exercise

For women with Polycystic Ovarian Syndrome (PCOS), weight gain is one of the most obvious and undesirable symptoms. You'll find it sneaking up on you until your pants won't button and your sleeves are stretched tightly over your arms.

The reason weight gain is so often a symptom of PCOS is because of the body's resistance, or lack of sensitivity, to insulin. Even though the pancreas is producing insulin as usual, the body reacts slowly or not at all, to the insulin. Insulin triggers the body to process the glucose, or blood sugar, for energy. When insulin isn't being recognized, then glucose isn't being used for energy. The glucose remains in the blood stream, meaning the pounds begin to add on, and you are at an increased risk for diabetes due to the chronic high levels of blood sugar.

Exercising regularly will help you prevent added poundage. Not only that, but exercising can help you avoid the related issues that can often accompany PCOS: high blood pressure and diabetes. Each of these conditions is caused by an abnormality with glucose levels and insulin absorption and production. Also, although it isn't a guarantee, regular exercise can also help you maintain regular periods. Women with PCOS may find that their menstruation cycles become irregular, or they may skip their periods altogether. Exercise may help you to stay on a normal cycle.

In this report, we'll delve into the best types of exercise for women with PCOS. We'll conclude with the value of proper nutrition. Exercise and nutrition go hand-in-hand. You won't be able to be truly healthy with one but not the other. Finally, we'll introduce you to some of our tastiest, healthiest recipes. These recipes have a low glycemic index, meaning their levels of sugar will affect your insulin levels less than foods with a high glycemic index.

Ready...Set...Go! Planning to Exercise Wisely

Exercise is the key to maintaining a healthy weight with PCOS. Because PCOS causes your body to process sugar differently than other women's bodies, you'll need to stick diligently to your exercise program for real results.

Getting started will first take setting goals. The best goals are S.M.A.R.T., meaning they are specific, measurable, actionable, realistic, and timely. You'll want to set a goal that specifically states how much weight you want to lose, or what your BMI (body mass index) will be. It needs to be measurable, so that later you can see how close you are to meeting your goal. It must be actionable, meaning you can take steps to reach it, such as exercising and eating a balanced diet. It absolutely needs to be realistic; consult your doctor, nutritionist or trainer to see if your weight-goal is reasonable. You'll only set yourself up for failure if you set a goal that is too intense. Working to reach your goal will take time and consistent discipline, but it's worth it for a healthy body! Finally, your goal should be timely. This means your goal will only be effective if you also put a time-goal on it.

Here is an example of an effective, measurable goal that will be realistic for some women with PCOS:

Example: "I will exercise for 120 minutes per week to lose 5 pounds by the last day of this month."

You'll see that this goal is specific, mentioning the exact amount of exercise, and that it is timely as well as measurable. For most people, it is also realistic. It's healthy to lose 1-2 pounds or less per week. Any more than that and you are putting severe strain on your body.

One of the traps people fall into when they concentrate on a weight goal is either over-exercising and/or under-eating. Over-exercising can result in burnout, meaning you will not feel motivated to work out. It can also cause injuries such as muscle tears, sprains, and severe fatigue. It's best to start out with a manageable exercise goal, and then build up incrementally each week. Your doctor or trainer can suggest options for you to track your progress and build up wisely.

Under-eating is also an obstacle to reaching your weight goal. By eating too little, you rob your body of necessary energy to exercise and build muscle. You aren't taking in enough nutrients and minerals for healthy hair, skin and overall health. Not only that, but if you eat fewer than 1200 calories per day, you run the risk of putting your body into starvation mode. This condition means your body's metabolism slows down, because it begins to conserve nutrients, believing you are in danger of starving. A slower metabolism means your body will burn fewer calories, and your rate of losing weight will drop dramatically.

All in all, it's best to increase your rate of exercise gradually while maintaining a healthy diet of fruits, vegetables, lean proteins, and whole grains. Set a goal that will allow you to do those activities without over-exercising or under-eating.

Building Your Endurance Step by Step, Rep by Rep

Rome wasn't built in a day; actually, it's still being constructed today as it constantly changes!

Your health is the same way. Living a healthy lifestyle takes time, and it is a lifelong pursuit. You'll be rewarded along the way with a great-looking body, toned muscles, and health benefits such as improved circulation and lower risk of heart disease and Alzheimer's disease. Rather than viewing it as a single task to accomplish, view exercise as lifelong habits you are making.

If you aren't currently active, start small. Everyone has to start somewhere. If you haven't been jogging lately, running a marathon will only exhaust your body, cause you injuries, and damage your resolve. Instead, start with manageable goals. For example, start at a weight level that is challenging for you after about five or six repetitions, or reps. Then, after two weeks at that same weight level, add two pounds. You'll find that you can manage it, and you'll become stronger over time.

Even a small amount of exercise can hold tremendous benefits for you. Research has shown that older people who exercised just once a day are 40% less likely to die than people at the same age who sit and do not exercise in any form.

Daily actions can make a big difference. Try making small changes, such as taking the stairs instead of the elevator. Go outside and walk your dog briskly. Or, if you don't have a canine companion, join up with a neighbor who walks their dog. When watching TV, get up during every commercial to move around. You can even try doing jumping jacks, squats, lunges or sit-ups during the commercials of your favorite show.

To burn fat

Make sure you are doing cardio in your target fat-burning zone. Your target fat-burning zone is the rate at which your heart is beating optimally. You will burn fat more effectively when you are exercising at this level than if you are overexerting yourself or under-exerting yourself. Your target zone is based on your Target Heart Rate, or THR, which you can find using the formula below:

226 – your age x .6 = Target Heart Rate

For example, if you are 35, your target heart rate is 226 – 35 x .6, which equals 114.6. This means your heart rate should be at about 114 or 115 when you are exercising, and that means you are gaining maximum fat burn. Hooray! Now, how can you test your heart rate to see how fast it is pumping? Many modern treadmills will tell you your heart-rate if you squeeze the bars for a few seconds on the metal plates provided, but a heart-rate monitor is likely to be even more accurate. You can purchase a heart-rate monitor at your local supermarket or department store, Target for example carries a good range.

To Lose or Maintain…That is the Question

If you are battling weight-gain with PCOS, it's going to take effort on your part to remove that weight and have it stay off.

Cardio at four to five times a week for 45 minutes per session is generally accepted as a powerful way to burn fat and keep it off. For maintenance, you'll be fine with two to three sessions of cardio ranging from 30 to 45 minutes as well.

Not everyone can start out at that level of intensity and frequency – in fact, most women need to start at a lower level. Do what's right for you, and write out a plan to gradually build up your level.

Starter Exercise Regiment

For a woman with PCOS, sometimes it's hard to know where to begin. Here is a great exercise regimen for a beginner to intermediate exerciser. You can adjust the weight-levels and minutes of cardio to suit your level of fitness. In general, follow these principles:

- Strength-train two times per week.

- Raise your weights by 2 pounds every other week.

- Strive for 90 to 120 minutes of cardio weekly.

- When performing strength-training, exhale when you are exerting and inhale when resting. For example, during bicep curls, breathe out when you are pulling the weights in, and breathe in when you are letting them down.

For those who are new to strength-training, here is a brief guide to some of the machines you'll be using:

Chest Press

Set the seat to a height at which you would be sitting with knees bent comfortably at 90 degrees. Select a weight that is challenging but doable. Sit straight up and place your head against the back of the seat. Grip the handles with palms facing down. Tighten your abdominal muscles, and press the handles forward until your elbows are mostly straight. Do NOT lock your elbows, however, but rather keep them slightly bent. Breathe out as you press them forward, then breathe in as you slowly allow them to come back toward you.

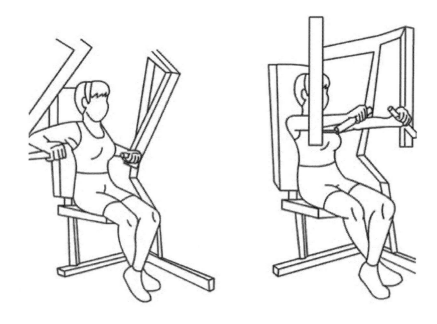

WomensRepublic.com

Push-Up

Kneel on the floor. Place your hands in front of you, palms down, a little wider than the width of your shoulders. For beginners, keep your knees on the floor, straighten your back, and lean on your arms until your nose almost touches the floor.

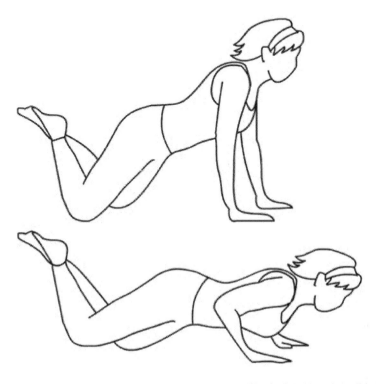

For intermediates, straighten your legs out behind you and rest on your toes. Complete a push-up by lowering yourself nearly to the floor, then pushing upwards to come back to your starting position. Exhale as you come back up. Keep your back straight. Do not lock your elbows in either position, but keep them at a slight bend.

Lateral Pull-Down

Sit so your feet are flat on floor, with the knees are above ankles, and your back is straight. Set your weight at a challenging level. Grab the handles overhead, palms facing forward. Pull the handles down gradually, bending your elbows in toward your sides. Be sure to breathe out as you pull down.

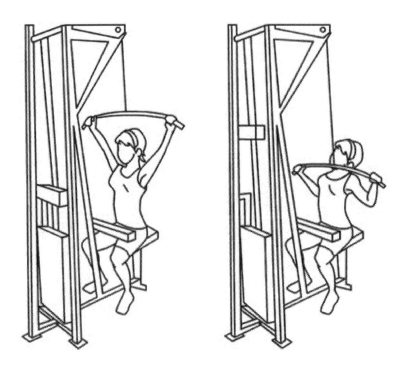

WomensRepublic.com

Crunches

Lay on your back on a mat or soft surface. Bend your knees and place your feet flat on the floor. Cross your arms in front of your chest. You can also place them behind your head, but you run the risk of pulling on your head and straining your neck.

Focus on your abdominal muscles, and pull forward, raising your shoulders and head off the ground. Inhale as you come up, exhale as you release and come down. Keep your head tucked in so your neck will not be sore later.

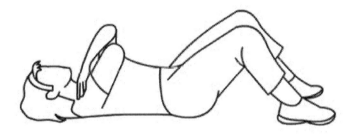

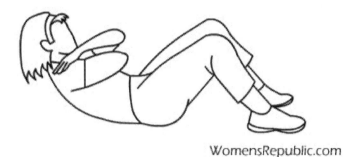

WomensRepublic.com

Squats

Stand with your feet slightly wider than your shoulders, and point your toes straight ahead. Lower your body slowly, bending at your hips. Keep your weight balanced on your heels, and keep your back as straight as possible. Keep your chest up.

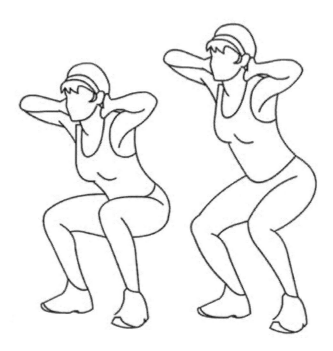

Lunges

While standing, step forward with one leg. Lower your body and bend both knees to a 90 degree angle. Do not let your knees go over your toes. Check between your feet to see that there is about 2 to 2.5 feet of space. Keep your weight on your front heel. Push back on your front heel to return to a standing position. Then switch legs.

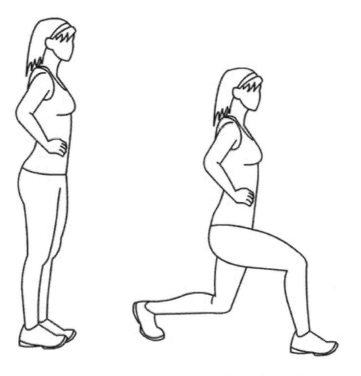

Bicycles

Lie on your back, and place your hands behind your ears. Stretch legs out so they are parallel to the floor. Then, pull your left knee in so that it is over your chest. Reach your right elbow up to touch or nearly touch your left knee over your chest. Then relax your leg and elbow back to the starting position. Repeat with the right knee and left elbow.

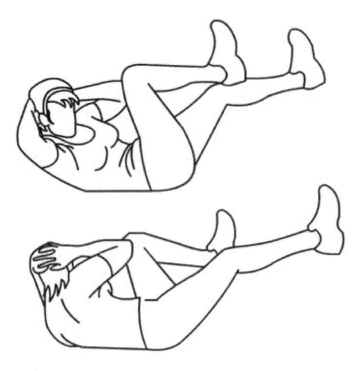

WomensRepublic.com

Plank

To make a plank, get into push-up position. Place your forearms on the floor and toes on the ground, then straighten out your back. Keep your feet together or only an inch apart. Focus on your abdominal muscles, and hold this position for 30 seconds.

Now that you are familiar with some of the types of exercise, focus on setting up a regular exercise routine for each day of the week.

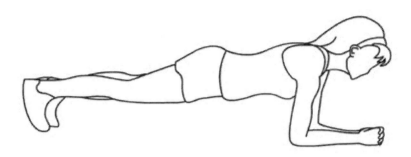

WomensRepublic.com

MONDAY: Stretch your arm, back and leg muscles before beginning. Start your week off right with intense, short bursts of cardio. Go for 5 minutes of walking at a comfortable speed, then 5 minutes at a brisk pace, then 5 minutes at a jog, then back to 5 minutes at a brisk pace, and 5 minutes of walking.

TUESDAY: It's strength-training day! Walk briskly for five minutes to get your heart rate up. This will make your strength-training more effective. Start out with arm exercises:

Arm exercises:

Chest press – 2 sets of 10 reps

Bicep curls – 2 sets of 10 reps

Leg exercises:

Leg raise – 2 sets of 10 reps

10 lunges with light weights

10 squats

Back exercises:

Back row - 2 sets of 10 reps

Lateral pull-downs – 2 sets of 10 reps

2 30-second planks

Abdominal exercises:

20 crunches

20 bicycles

10 push-ups (You can rest on your knees if you are just starting push-ups.)

WEDNESDAY: It's hump-day, and we'll crest the middle of the week by cracking down with some cardio! Complete a set of 20 jumping-jacks. Warm up by walking briskly for 5 minutes. Then do 10 minutes at a jogging pace. Slow to a brisk walk for 5 minutes, then go back to another 10 minute jog. When you are finished with that, stretch well so that you won't be as sore afterwards.

THURSDAY: Strength-training day #2 is here! Be sure to do your 5-minute brisk walk as a warm-up before starting. Follow the same exercises as you did on Tuesday. Keep your weights at the same level.

FRIDAY: Light cardio. Warm up for 5 minutes. Jog for 15 minutes at a comfortable pace. Try a new gait, such as high-knees or butt-kicks for 5 minutes apiece. Be sure you stretch your legs well.

SATURDAY: Try a new cardio exercise, such as taking a hike, swimming, bicycling or dancing! Go to a Zumba class with friends. Make today about a fresh, fun way to exercise!

SUNDAY: REST DAY! Soak in a hot bath or get a massage. You deserve it! Plus, your rest will allow your body to recover for the next week.

Keep It Fresh 'n Fun

Stay motivated by varying the types of exercise you do. Go for Zumba one day, jogging the next day, jumping rope and then swimming after that. Finding an exercise buddy or selecting a regular class to attend will go a long way. Not only will your exercise be more fun with friends, but they'll also hold you accountable. Decorate your walls, car and desk with positive, motivational pictures or posters.

As you achieve your milestones which you set earlier in your exercise plan, reward yourself. Now, we're not talking about detrimental rewards, such as cupcakes and candy, but other types of rewards. Think about seeing a movie, or buying a new outfit that shows off your trimmer figure. Spring for some new exercise threads or hair accessories. Or simply reward yourself with some quality time relaxing, such as a massage or luxuriously long soak in a hot tub. Your body will thank you, your mind will be reinvigorated, and you'll be firmly on the right track to continue on your way to a healthy body!

More Effective Fat-Burning: Your Target Heart Rate

Why walk for long, slow hours if you can run for an intense burst and burn the same level of calories? You can jump-start your way to burning calories by raising your intensity level safely.

When you exercise, your heart is pumping oxygenated blood to your muscles to keep them going like the Energizer Bunny. From the lowest heart-rate zone to the highest zone, you are giving your body invaluable benefits, such as a lowered blood pressure, reduced cholesterol, and of course, fat-burn. The sweat is worth it!

Let's look at the zones so you can see where you need to be. The best way to check and see if you are in your preferred zone as you exercise is by using a heart monitor.

Healthy Heart Zone – 50-60% of your maximum heart rate. This zone is great if you are just returning to being active. You'll achieve all the benefits we just discussed and even lower your chance of degenerative diseases in the future, such as Alzheimer's. That's right – as your body stays fit, your mind is more likely to stay sharp! Plus, get ready for this: you burn 85% fat at this level. Eight-five percent is obviously a very high percentage, but the total amount of calories you burn may not be as high as another zone. So if you want to max your percentage and the total amounts, take a look at these other zones.

Fat-Burning Zone – 60-70% of your maximum heart rate. The raised intensity level continues to burn your fat at 85% but burns more total calories. That's a win-win!

Aerobic Zone – 70-80% of your maximum heart rate. You are working on your endurance at this zone. Your heart will become stronger, allowing you to perform at a higher level. You'll burn 50% from fat.

Anaerobic Zone – 80-90% of your maximum heart rate. Wow, you are an athlete! At this rate, you are burning up oxygen at the highest level you can during exercise. In future workouts, you'll resist fatigue better and be able to work out for a longer period of time. You don't burn as many calories from fat, however – just 15%.

Maximum Heart Rate – 90-100% of your heart rate. Competing in the Olympics? Sprinting for a gold medal? You are working as hard as your heart will allow and burning the highest number of calories. Be careful of going at this intensity. Many who are not trained athletes can injure their bodies and overwork their heart. Save this for the races when it counts.

Each of these rates has a right time and place, depending on your exercise routine. Switch it up for a stronger heart and more effective workout. Remember to pace yourself and build up gradually so you can work out longer and burn more calories from fat.

Now that you know the various levels of heart rate intensity and how that helps you burn fat, how can you raise your metabolic rate? See the next article on raising your metabolic rate to find out.

Raise Your Metabolic Rate

Raise your rate! Your metabolic rate, that is. PCOS will still be with you, but you'll have a powerful weapon to help keep you trim and fit: your metabolism.

When you increase the rate at which you burn calories, your workouts will be more effective.

Yes, as you grow older, your metabolism slows down. When you don't burn off the calories you've consumed, they are converted into fat for later use. With PCOS, it's harder to get these fat cells to burn, as your body is less sensitive to insulin. But there are many small, daily actions you can take to raise your metabolism and then let your body burn calories even when you're resting. Think about that: you can actually burn calories as you sit or sleep!

Key pointers for boosting that magic ratio:

EAT FREQUENT SMALL MEALS. Yes, eat more often! You probably didn't think you'd hear that in your plan to lose weight. You can eat more often, but the key is smaller portion size. Instead of a sandwich and fruit cup at lunch, try having the sandwich at lunch time and the fruit two to three hours later. What this means is your stomach will be constantly engaging in digestive processes that yes, use energy which means using calories. Make your stomach work! Just be sure that the foods you are consuming are not high in caloric content – choose wisely from among fruits, veggies, lean meats and low fat dairy products.

PACK A HEALTHY SNACK. Snacks like fruit, raisins, nuts and oats can ease your hunger pangs, boost your energy and even raise your metabolism. Go crazy with the Craisins!

DRINK ICED WATER. You make your body work that much harder when you drink cool to cold water. It actually has to expend energy to heat up the water, which means more calories are used up.

EXERCISE AT THE RIGHT HEART RATE. If you read the previous article on your target heart rate, you know that exercising at 60-70% of your maximum heart rate can burn up to 85% of calories from fat. Sustain your exercise at that level for 30 to 45 minutes per day, and you'll be burning calories and boosting your metabolism.

LIFT WEIGHTS. You may have heard that muscle burns more calories than fat does. Long after you lift weights, your muscle cells are still burning calories. They burn calories even when you're asleep!

MOVE. That's right, one of the best things you can do is simply to move. Go for the stairs instead of the elevator. Volunteer to go to the store and choose to carry a basket instead of a grocery cart. Take small walks on your break during work. Squeeze your butt and thighs while sitting in the car for long periods of time. Do lunges, crunches or jog in-place while you watch TV commercials. Every move you do means a fitter you!

Eat Smart, Live Well

If you have been diagnosed with PCOS, your menu will need to look a little different. Fill your plate with lean proteins, fruits, vegetable, and whole grain. Green vegetables such as cabbage, celery, spinach, broccoli, green beans, artichokes and asparagus provide your body with antioxidants that boost your body's immunity.

You'll want to avoid unnecessary, processed fats and sugars, such as candy and fried foods. Lowering the amount of blood sugar you intake means you're helping to keep glucose levels down which, when high, cause your ovaries to work overtime and your fat cells to keep the fat inside instead of burning it. It's okay to give yourself a break every now and then, but remember to balance it out with exercise.

Keep your dairy intake low. Yogurts are a healthy source of dairy, but butter, milk, and cheese carry significant fats. Try low-fat or non-dairy substitutes. Even when cooking, replace butter with margarine or nonfat cooking spray.

As for beverages, keep H2O in your bottle. Water will keep you hydrated, giving you energy to complete your workout. You can use calorie-free flavor agents, such as Crystal Light or Mio, but be cautious of those that come laden with sugar. Check the package to be sure you're getting great taste without the burden for your waist.

Special workout drinks meant to replenish electrolytes can be excellent for supporting a high level of energy and hydration before, during and after workouts. However, be cautious of the kinds you buy. Check the labels first to see what added sugars there are. You'll find certain brands include massive quantities of calories that will make you see slower progress in weight-loss.

It's a hard truth, but alcohol is filled with empty calories. If you are serious about maintaining a healthy weight, you'll want to lower your intake. Not only are the calories problematic, but the nature of alcohol in relaxing you and lowering your inhibitions means you'll be more likely to start munching on those chicken wings and cheese fries on the table. You'll make poorer choices and betray your hard work on the tread mill. If you like your liquor too much to give it up, then select smaller serving sizes and types of beverages that do not contain mass amounts of sugar.

You'll find that by following these simple rules, you can increase your weight loss and the overall health of your body. One of the best rules you can follow is selecting foods based on how they rank according to the glycemic index.

What is the glycemic index, you ask?

If you've been diagnosed with PCOS, and you haven't heard of the glycemic index, it's time to introduce you properly.

The glycemic index is a powerful tool for helping you lose weight, maintain a healthy weight, and prevent weight gain. Created in the 1980s, the glycemic index was originally designed to help diabetic people manage their blood sugar. At its core, the glycemic index is simply a scientific method of measuring the impact that specific foods will have on your blood sugar levels. You probably already knew that a chocolate doughnut will raise your blood sugar more than celery, for example.

Like the judges on American Idol, the glycemic index ranks foods. Foods can be labeled on a scale of 0 to 100 on how rapidly they raise your blood sugar. If your blood sugar is going to rocket sky-high, the food will have a higher score. If the type of food will take time to affect your glucose, its score will be lower on the scale.

In general, if a food has a score of 55 or less, that's low. If it's between 56 and 69, that's pretty average. And if its glycemic index is 70 or more, you probably should avoid it.

When you are calculating the total glycemic index of your meal, that's called a glycemic load. Not the most clever name, but it works. You generally want to keep your daily glycemic load under 100.

Here's the magic formula for finding the glycemic load:

glycemic index of food x number of grams of carbs ÷ 100 = glycemic load

For example, if a slice of white bread has a glycemic index of 70, take 70 and multiply it by how many grams of carbohydrates it has. The grams of carbohydrates can be found on the package, so say it is 15 grams. 70 times 15 equals 1,050, then divided by 100 for a glycemic load score of 10.5.

The glycemic index has become an important nutritional tool for women with PCOS. If you would like to try managing your blood sugar with the help of the glycemic index, consider searching for the glycemic index of your food on a mobile app, web site, or purchasing a book on the glycemic index. You can find web sites such as GlycemicGourmet.com, GlycemicIndex.com, or a mobile app such as Glycemic Index Meal Planner.

It may seem like a pain to calculate your food, but it's far more effective for you than carb-counting. For example, one cup of dark cherries and one cup of corn each contain around 15 carbohydrates, give or take. But the blood sugar levels for each are vastly different: those cherries are ranked with a 63 glycemic index, and the corn is only a 48. Because PCOS means your body will be greatly affected by higher levels of blood sugar, you need to aim for those foods with a lower glycemic index. You won't know the better foods for you by looking at the carb count on the nutrition label.

You'll find that using the glycemic index helps you manage your blood sugar, which prevents weight gain. If you keep your blood sugar from rising, your body will produce less insulin, and your muscles can use the insulin more effectively.

Low Glycemic Diet for PCOS

Having read the previous section, you now know about the weight loss and healthy weight maintenance that can come from following the glycemic index. If you are woman with PCOS, you need to focus on regulating your blood sugar, since your body is less sensitive to insulin, which would normally cause that blood sugar to be used up as energy. Lots of blood sugar means lots of weight gain

So, using the glycemic index to select healthy, satisfying foods that will fill you up and keep blood sugar down is key to preventing bulge. Here are some of the guidelines to a low glycemic diet:

- Select foods from the lower end of the glycemic index table which have high levels of nutrients.

- Limit your carbohydrates. Aim to have 40-50% of your calories from carbs. Most people's diets give them 60% of their calories from carbohydrates, but as a woman with PCOS, you're better off with fewer carbohydrates.

- Eat smaller meals throughout the day, rather than three large ones. This will help you avoid blood sugar spikes after you eat and valleys in-between meals.

- Snack on proteins, like nuts, or another healthy fat source, like avocado.

It's important to understand that using the glycemic index does not mean that you should never eat foods with higher glycemic index scores. You can eat them on occasion if the portion size is minimal. You might be surprised by some foods that have higher effects on your blood sugar, such as potatoes. There are many positive benefits to a food like potatoes, such as potassium, vitamin C, vitamin B6, and more. Just be sure to couple this food with proteins and other low glycemic indexed foods.

Be sure to check the glycemic index of foods before automatically assuming they have a high score. Some will surprise you. Coca-Cola, for example, has a score of 53, because its high fructose corn syrup actually has a low glycemic index (but many people believe high fructose corn syrup is horrible for your health, some discretion is advised), too. Pound cake, bananas, macaroni, instant chocolate pudding, and others are great treats for you, because they won't wreck your blood sugar levels. Just be sure you are keeping them within a reasonable portion size, because the calories and carbohydrates are still considerable, the more you serve.

It's normal that foods contain carbohydrates, and you need them in the right quantities. Your body uses carbohydrates to convert into energy. By using the glycemic index, you can select those foods which will give you the energy you need without the severely high level of glucose. As a woman with PCOS, planning out your meals in advance will probably help you to stick to your weight loss plans and skip the sugary snags.

Lean Meats and Low-Fat Dairy Treats

Moooove over, dairy and fatty meats. We women with PCOS are taking charge of our health and avoiding the pitfalls of foods that create weight gain.

For women with PCOS, our optimal diet is low in saturated fats, low in carbohydrates, moderate in proteins, and as low a glycemic index as possible. Our plates should often look as though they were fresh out of a garden: fresh vegetables, colorful fruits, legumes, and whole grains.

But we all crave savory burgers, chicken wraps and tasty fish from time to time! Red meats give you protein, iron, and calcium. So what's a girl with PCOS to do to avoid those carbs?

Interestingly enough, meat doesn't contain carbohydrates! That's right: chicken, fish, pork, beef, steak – no carbs at all. That means that they are considered outside of the glycemic index. Keep the portion sizes small though, and avoid breading them or adding cracker crumbs. The style of preparation is where the additional carbs come in, with breading, frying, cooking in oil or butter, and other fattening methods that add carbs to the meat.

Fish are fantastic sources of health benefits for your body that you might not get otherwise. The oilier the fish, the more omega-3 fatty acids it contains, which helps your body to reduce inflammation and blood clotting and lower your risk of heart disease. Get this: eating fish just one time per week can lower your risk of a fatal heart attack by forty percent! Again, you want to select oily fish, such as swordfish, salmon, tuna, perch, mackerel, and sardines. But remember not to select those that are prepared with fattening vegetable oil, because that's where the extra carbs sneak their way in. Instead, go for those that are marinated, grilled, or fried with canola oil.

Dairy can be quite contrary. But if you select low-fat options, you're saving your body a lot of trouble. Look for fat-free milk and yogurt, because these provide you with calcium and Vitamin D. Their low glycemic index score doesn't hurt, either.

In fact, dairy products, like red meat, provide that much-needed source of calcium for women's bodies. They contain protein, Vitamin B12, zinc, and much more. With a low-fat version or soy milk substitute, you may want to select a product where these vitamins have been added. For example, there are omega-3 enriched eggs that contain much higher levels of those omega-3s than regular eggs.

Get out there and marinate and grill some lean meat! Don't be afraid to include dairy products in your diet, so long as they are low in fat and high in vitamins! You'll feel better and still have those flavors you love.

What's On the Menu: Recipes for Women with PCOS

In the next section are recipes with a low glycemic index. These recipes taste delicious and will satisfy you and your family. They'll keep you on-track with maintaining a healthy weight and avoiding the weight-gain that can come with PCOS.

Try the following recipes today. You'll find that your taste buds are happy, your body will be healthy, and you'll look in the mirror proudly.

RECAP Glycemic Load:

The Glycemic Load is the easiest way to keep a check on our weight and it is easily calculated by multiplying a food's Glycemic Index (as a percentage) by the number of net carbohydrates in a given serving.

Glycemic Load gives an idea about the rise in blood-sugar levels with the consumption of the concerned food.

GL = GI/100 x Net Carbohydrates

A GL of 20 or more is high, a GL of 11 to 19 inclusive is medium, and a GL of 10 or less is low.

Smoothies

1. Banana and Strawberry Smoothie

Preparation time	5 minutes
Ready time	10 minutes
Serves	2
Serving quantity/unit	260mL/8.8fl oz
Glycemic index/serving	45 ±3
Glycemic Load/serving	11
Calories	140 Cal
Total Fat	0.7 g
Cholesterol	0 mg
Sodium	3 mg
Total Carbohydrates	35.2 g
Dietary fibers	5.2g
Sugars	19.7 g
Protein	2 g
Vitamin C	123%
Vitamin A	4%
Iron	12%
Calcium	2%

Ingredients

- 2 Bananas sliced
- 1 1/2 cup strawberries
- Ice cubes

Method

- Peel the banana and slice it.
- Add the washed strawberries and bananas into a blender and add ice cubes.
- Run the blender at medium for a minute and serve the smoothie chilled.

TIP: This smoothie is ideal for a refreshing start in the mornings and it is low in Glycemic Index and has a low Glycemic load too, which helps to maintain a healthy lifestyle.

2. Vegetable Smoothie

Preparation time	5 minutes
Ready time	10 minutes
Serves	2
Serving quantity/unit	236mL/8 fl oz
Glycemic index/serving	40±3
Glycemic Load/serving	5
Calories	70 Cal
Total Fat	0.7 g
Cholesterol	0 mg
Sodium	55 mg
Total Carbohydrates	16.4 g
Dietary fibers	4.8g
Sugars	9.4 g
Protein	2.8g
Vitamin C	60%
Vitamin A	245%
Iron	5%
Calcium	5%

Ingredients

- 4 Tomatoes chopped
- 2 carrots
- 2 capsicum
- Salt and Pepper to taste
- 1 teaspoon lemon juice
- 1 teaspoon ginger juice
- 2 sprigs of mint leaves
- Ice cubes

Method

- Wash the vegetables and chop them roughly.
- Add them in a blender along with the lemon and ginger juice.
- Add salt and pepper and mix till a smooth blend is formed.
- Serve chilled with ice cubes.

TIP: Vegetables provide complete nutrition so this smoothie is an asset for people who want to lose weight. Freshly made Vegetable Smoothie tastes the best.

Snacks

3. Potato Crisps

Preparation time	15 minutes
Ready time	35 minutes
Serves	20 Pieces
Serving quantity/unit	50 G / 1.8 ounce
Glycemic index/serving	55±3
Glycemic Load/serving	10
Calories	76 Cal
Total Fat	1.5 g
Cholesterol	0 mg
Sodium	3 mg
Total Carbohydrates	11.5 g
Dietary fibers	1.2g
Sugars	0.5 g
Protein	1.4g
Vitamin C	14%
Vitamin A	0%
Iron	3%
Calcium	0%

Ingredients

- 4 potatoes
- Oil to fry
- 1 cup all-purpose flour
- Salt and pepper to taste

Method

- Peel the potatoes and cut wedges out of them and soak in water.
- In a plastic bag add the salt, pepper and flour them with a tissue paper.
- Mix them with the flour and spices in the bag shaking thoroughly.
- Heat oil in a pan and deep fry the wedges.
- Serve hot with sauce.

TIP: The potatoes can be cut in the shape of cubes or French fries. Spices can be varied as per individual choice.

4. Apricot Cookies

Preparation time	20 minutes
Ready time	50 minutes
Serves	24
Serving quantity/unit	30 G/1.05 ounce
Glycemic index/serving	47±4
Glycemic Load/serving	8
Calories	124 Cal
Total Fat	4.2 g
Cholesterol	17 mg
Sodium	39 mg
Total Carbohydrates	21.4 g
Dietary fibers	0g
Sugars	2.4 g
Protein	1.8g
Vitamin C	0%
Vitamin A	3%
Iron	5%
Calcium	3%

Ingredients

- 3 cups All-purpose flour
- 1 tablespoon baking powder
- 1/3 cup sugar
- Pinch of Salt
- 1/4 teaspoon cardamom powder
- 1/2 cup melted butter
- 1 cup apricot syrup
- 1 egg

Method

- Preheat the oven to 350 degrees.
- Mix sugar, flour, baking powder, salt along with cardamom powder.
- Add butter to this mixture.
- Add apricot syrup and eggs and mix well.
- Knead the dough softly.
- Cool it for some time in the refrigerator.
- Make the dough into a 1/4 inch thick roll.
- Cut the dough with a cookie cutter.

- Bake the cookies for around 10 to 12 minutes till they turn golden brown.
- Let them cool and store in an airtight container.

TIP: Sugar coated cookies amount to a higher GI Load hence should be avoided.

5. Herbs Crackers

Preparation time	15 minutes
Ready time	35 minutes
Serves	12
Serving quantity/unit	25G/0.8 ounce
Glycemic index/serving	52±8
Glycemic Load/serving	9
Calories	106 Cal
Total Fat	7.8 g
Cholesterol	20 mg
Sodium	55 mg
Total Carbohydrates	8.0 g
Dietary fibers	0g
Sugars	0 g
Protein	1.2g
Vitamin C	0%
Vitamin A	5%
Iron	3%
Calcium	0%

Ingredients

- 1 cup all-purpose flour
- 1/4 teaspoon pepper
- 1/2 teaspoon dried herbs powder
- 1/4 cup water
- 1/2 cup butter

Method

- Preheat oven at 400 degree.
- Combine all the ingredients in a blender and pulse.
- Add a little more water if needed.
- Form a dough and let it stand for 10 minutes.
- Roll the dough in a sheet of 1/8th inch and transfer it to a cookie sheet.
- Cut the shape of cookies as desired.

- Bake the cookies for 10 to 12 minutes till slightly brown.
- Remove the cookies and let them cool.
- Transfer in an airtight container.

TIP: The herbs can be replaced with cinnamon powder or with 1/2 teaspoon of garlic paste to make cinnamon or garlic cookies respectively.

Breakfast

6. Pancakes made with coconut flour

Preparation time	10 minutes
Ready time	25 minutes
Serves	12
Serving quantity/unit	96G/3.4oz
Glycemic index/serving	46±3
Glycemic Load/serving	11
Calories	213 Cal
Total Fat	8.3 g
Cholesterol	27mg
Sodium	174 mg
Total Carbohydrates	19g
Dietary fibers	10g
Sugars	4.4g
Protein	5.1g
Vitamin C	16%
Vitamin A	1%
Iron	1%
Calcium	1%

Ingredients

- 1/4 cup coconut oil
- 2 eggs
- 3 dates deseeded
- 4 tablespoon thick orange juice
- 3 cups coconut flour
- 1 teaspoon baking soda
- 1 cup Strawberries chopped

Method

- Mix the coconut oil well with eggs and orange pulp.
- Blend this mixture with flour and other ingredients except strawberries and make a smooth batter.
- Now heat a skillet for making the pancakes. If you have a griddle for pancakes then it is better.
- Add the chopped strawberries in the batter and mix properly with a ladle.
- Pour the batter on the skillet taking 1/2 cup at a time and making pancakes of about 3 inches diameter.
- Cook one side till done and then flip on the other side and cook for around 3 to 5 minutes.
- Serve with nuts or sliced fruits.

TIP: The pancakes must be cooked till slight brown from both sides. Be careful not to overcook or burn the pancakes.

7. Low-fat Yoghurt with fruit

Preparation time	5 minutes
Ready time	10 minutes
Serves	2
Serving quantity/unit	150G/5.3oz
Glycemic index/serving	31±8
Glycemic Load/serving	9
Calories	83 Cal
Total Fat	7.8 g
Cholesterol	20 mg
Sodium	55 mg
Total Carbohydrates	8.0 g
Dietary fibers	0g
Sugars	0 g
Protein	1.2g
Vitamin C	0%
Vitamin A	5%
Iron	3%
Calcium	0%

Ingredients

- 2 cups whipped, low fat yoghurt
- 1/2 cup chopped strawberry
- 1/4 cup chopped wild berries

- Salt and Pepper to taste

Method

- Whisk the yoghurt in a blender.
- Take a serving bowl and add the fruit in it.
- Sprinkle salt and pepper.
- Mix the fruits with the yoghurt and garnish with mint leaves.
- Serve chilled.

TIP: Fruits can be fresh or canned too, but should be chopped in small cubes to make the yoghurt appetizing.

8. Oats Porridge

Preparation time	10 minutes
Ready time	25 minutes
Serves	4
Serving quantity/unit	200G/7.1oz
Glycemic index/serving	58±8
Glycemic Load/serving	12
Calories	106 Cal
Total Fat	1.7 g
Cholesterol	2mg
Sodium	601 mg
Total Carbohydrates	20 g
Dietary fibers	2.1g
Sugars	6.1 g
Protein	3.6g
Vitamin C	0%
Vitamin A	1%
Iron	5%
Calcium	5%

Ingredients

- 1 cup oats
- 2 1/2 cup water
- 1 teaspoon salt
- 1 tablespoon honey
- 1/2 teaspoon cardamom powder
- 1/2 cup low fat milk

Method

- Mix the oats, water, honey, cardamom in a pan and bring to a boil.
- Simmer the oats stirring continuously for 5 minutes.
- Remove from heat and pour in bowls.
- Add little milk in each bowl and serve.

TIP: The porridge can be garnished with chopped fruits like apple or strawberries

9. Fruit and Muesli bread

Preparation time	70 minutes
Ready time	120 minutes
Serves	24
Serving quantity/unit	30G/1.1oz
Glycemic index/serving	53±4
Glycemic Load/serving	7
Calories	109 Cal
Total Fat	1.6 g
Cholesterol	0 mg
Sodium	5 mg
Total Carbohydrates	18.3 g
Dietary fibers	3.8g
Sugars	0.9g
Protein	3.9g
Vitamin C	0%
Vitamin A	0%
Iron	5%
Calcium	1%

Ingredients

- 8 cups water
- 2 tablespoons oil
- 3 cups broken wheat
- 1 tablespoon honey
- 1/4 cup low-fat milk
- 1/2 cup muesli with fruit
- 2 tablespoon instant yeast

Method

- Knead all the ingredients into a semi-hard dough.
- Cover with a permeable cloth and keep for 1/2 an hour.
- Add water to the bread maker.
- Add the dough into the bucket and fit the bucket into the bread maker.
- Set the program of the bread maker as instructed.
- Remove the bread when ready and let it stand.
- Leave the loaf for an hour and the cut into the desired size and serve.

TIP: This bread can be eaten without applying anything. Apply jam or honey and serve.

10. Sweet corn on the cob

Preparation time	5 minutes
Ready time	10 minutes
Serves	6
Serving quantity/unit	80G/2.8oz
Glycemic index/serving	48±2
Glycemic Load/serving	8
Calories	58 Cal
Total Fat	2.8 g
Cholesterol	6 mg
Sodium	35 mg
Total Carbohydrates	11.9 g
Dietary fibers	1.3g
Sugars	04.3g
Protein	2.9g
Vitamin C	6%
Vitamin A	4%
Iron	1%
Calcium	5%

Ingredients

- 4 corn ears
- 1 cup of milk
- 2 cups water
- 1 teaspoon Sugar
- 1/2 tablespoon butter

Method

- Take a large pan and mix the milk water and sugar along with the butter.
- Bring to a boil and add the corn.
- Let it boil for around 7 to 8 minutes.
- Remove the corns with tongs and wrap with foil papers.
- Serve with lemon and salt.

TIP: The husks and silk of the corns should be removed before use. If the corns are too big they can be broken into two pieces as required.

11. Stuffed bun with shallots and meat

Preparation time	10 minutes
Ready time	30 minutes
Serves	4
Serving quantity/unit	120G/4.3oz
Glycemic index/serving	59±8
Glycemic Load/serving	14
Calories	276 Cal
Total Fat	10.2 g
Cholesterol	46 mg
Sodium	170 mg
Total Carbohydrates	18.3 g
Dietary fibers	0.6g
Sugars	1.8g
Protein	19.7g
Vitamin C	4%
Vitamin A	6%
Iron	11%
Calcium	5%

Ingredients

- 4 buns
- 250 gm boneless shredded meat boiled
- 100 g shallots
- 1 teaspoon garlic paste
- 2 tablespoons oil
- Salt and pepper to taste

Method

- Slit the buns from the middle and keep aside.
- Add oil to a pan and sauté the shallots.
- Add the garlic paste and stir.
- Sprinkle with salt and pepper and then add the boiled meat.
- Stir for 3 minutes and fry.
- Fill the above mix in the buns.
- Bake the buns for 5 minutes in a preheated oven at 150 degrees.
- Serve warm.

TIP: Meat can be replaced with carrots, beans and peas to get a veggie delight...

12. Baked beans in ham sauce

Preparation time	20 minutes
Ready time	180 minutes
Serves	8
Serving quantity/unit	150 G/5.3oz
Glycemic index/serving	53±4
Glycemic Load/serving	13
Calories	140 Cal
Total Fat	6.7 g
Cholesterol	82mg
Sodium	216 mg
Total Carbohydrates	10.4 g
Dietary fibers	3.3g
Sugars	3.5 g
Protein	31.1 g
Vitamin C	24%
Vitamin A	17%
Iron	12%
Calcium	4%

Ingredients

- 300g harlot beans
- 900 g smoked hock
- 4 teaspoon oil
- 1 onion chopped
- 800 g tomatoes, diced

- Salt and Pepper to taste

Method

- Soak the beans overnight in water.
- Place the beans and ham hock in a pan of water and simmer for 30 minutes.
- Remove the ham and beans and keep aside.
- Do not throw the liquid.
- Heat oil in a pan and cook the onion till brown.
- Add the tomatoes and liquid and bring to a boil.
- Shred the ham pieces and add them to the pan.
- Add the beans and simmer for another 30 minutes till the gravy thickens.
- Add salt and pepper and serve hot with bread.

TIP: The beans can be prepared in tomato sauce also without the ham hock.

Lunch

13. Black Eyed Beans

Preparation time	15 minutes
Ready time	60 minutes
Serves	2
Serving quantity/unit	150 G/5.3oz
Glycemic index/serving	33±4
Glycemic Load/serving	10
Calories	168 Cal
Total Fat	4.7 g
Cholesterol	0mg
Sodium	16 mg
Total Carbohydrates	30.4 g
Dietary fibers	11.3g
Sugars	4.2 g
Protein	10.1 g
Vitamin C	14%
Vitamin A	5%
Iron	17%
Calcium	4%

Ingredients

- 2 cups of black eyed beans

- 4 cups water
- 1 onion, chopped
- 1 teaspoon garlic paste
- 2 teaspoons oil
- 1 teaspoon ginger paste
- Red pepper 1/2 teaspoon
- 1 Tomato chopped
- Salt and Pepper to taste

Method

- Heat a pan and add oil. Sauté the onions in the oil.
- Add garlic and ginger paste.
- Stir and add salt and pepper and then add chopped tomato.
- Stir fry the black eyed beans and simmer for 50 minutes after adding sufficient water and covering.
- Remove the pan from heat and garnish with coriander leaves.

TIP: The Black Eyes beans should be soaked before cooking to get better results.

14. Mung Beans fried

Preparation time	15minutes
Ready time	60 minutes
Serves	2
Serving quantity/unit	150 G/ 5.3 oz
Glycemic index/serving	33±4
Glycemic Load/serving	10
Calories	150 Cal
Total Fat	8.7 g
Cholesterol	0mg
Sodium	36 mg
Total Carbohydrates	67.4 g
Dietary fibers	11.5g
Sugars	10.2g
Protein	25.3 g
Vitamin C	15%
Vitamin A	36%
Iron	19%
Calcium	34%

Ingredients

- 2 cups mung beans
- 1 onion, chopped
- 1 tablespoon oil
- 2 garlic cloves, paste
- 1 chili
- 1 tomato, chopped
- 1 teaspoon cumin seed
- Salt and Pepper to taste

Method

- Heat a pan and add oil.
- Add cumin seeds and after they splutter add the onions and sauté till slight brown.
- Add the garlic paste and tomatoes.
- Now stir in the mung and chili along with the salt and pepper.
- Stir for few minutes and then add water.
- Cover and simmer for around 20 minutes or till the mung becomes tender.
- Dry the remaining water and garnish with coriander leaves.
- Serve hot.

TIP: The mung can be sprouted and used in order to increase the protein content.

15. Chick Peas Hummus dip

Preparation time	5 minutes
Ready time	15 minutes
Serves	16
Serving quantity/unit	30 G/1.05oz
Glycemic index/serving	23±4
Glycemic Load/serving	3
Calories	120 Cal
Total Fat	3.7 g
Cholesterol	0mg
Sodium	6 mg
Total Carbohydrates	15.4 g
Dietary fibers	4.3g
Sugars	2.5 g
Protein	4.9 g
Vitamin C	3%
Vitamin A	1%
Iron	9%
Calcium	3%

Ingredients

- 2 cups boiled chickpeas
- 2 tablespoons sesame paste (tahini)
- 2 tablespoons lemon juice
- 2 garlic pods
- 2 tablespoon olive oil
- Sprig of mint

Method

- Drain the water from the boiled chickpeas.
- Add the chickpeas and garlic in the blender and mix.
- Add tahini, lemon juice, 1 tablespoon olive oil and mix again.
- Pour the mix in a serving bowl and add remaining olive oil.
- Garnish with mint leaves and serve.

TIP: This dip can be made and kept in the refrigerator for a week. Keep it well covered.

16. Mushroom and spinach Mix

Preparation time	45 minutes
Ready time	90 minutes
Serves	4
Serving quantity/unit	86 G/3.0oz
Glycemic index/serving	26±4
Glycemic Load/serving	11
Calories	85 Cal
Total Fat	7.0 g
Cholesterol	0mg
Sodium	116 mg
Total Carbohydrates	5.4 g
Dietary fibers	1.3g
Sugars	1.5 g
Protein	1.1 g
Vitamin C	20%
Vitamin A	56%
Iron	6%
Calcium	4%

Ingredients

- 1 onion, chopped
- 2 teaspoon garlic paste
- 2 tablespoon oil
- 4 cups spinach blanched
- 1 cup mushrooms chopped
- 1 teaspoon hot sauce
- 1 teaspoon Worcestershire sauce
- 1 cup vegetable stock
- Salt to taste

Method

- Heat oil in a pan and add the onion to sauté.
- Add the garlic paste and stir well.
- Put the chopped mushrooms and stir fry for 2 to 3 minutes and then add stock and simmer for 7 minutes after covering.
- Stir the mushrooms and add the sauces and spinach and let the vegetables simmer for few minutes.

- Serve hot with rice.

TIP: The spinach should be boiled with a pinch of sugar in order to retain its color.

17. Chicken Korma

Preparation time	10 minutes
Ready time	25 minutes
Serves	2
Serving quantity/unit	300 G/10.6oz
Glycemic index/serving	44±4
Glycemic Load/serving	10
Calories	340 Cal
Total Fat	10.7 g
Cholesterol	120mg
Sodium	209 mg
Total Carbohydrates	20.9 g
Dietary fibers	7.3g
Sugars	5.5 g
Protein	43.4 g
Vitamin C	37%
Vitamin A	23%
Iron	22%
Calcium	15%

Ingredients

- 1 onion
- 2 cloves garlic
- 10 cloves
- 10 cardamoms
- 2 cinnamon sticks
- 2 chicken breasts
- 1/2 teaspoon coriander powder
- 1/2 teaspoon cumin powder
- 2 tomatoes(sliced)
- Salt to taste

Method

- Heat oil in a pan and cook the cloves, cinnamon, cardamom in a pan.
- Stir in onion and garlic and sauté.

- Add the chicken breasts and cook for 5 to 7 minutes.
- Season with coriander, cumin and salt and add the tomatoes and stir for 2 minutes.
- Add water and simmer for around 10 minutes.
- Serve hot after garnishing with parsley.

TIP: Chicken Korma is tastes best when served with Peshawar rice or butter Nan.

18. Basmati white rice with Green peas

Preparation time	10 minutes
Ready time	50 minutes
Serves	8
Serving quantity/unit	150 G/5.3oz
Glycemic index/serving	43±4
Glycemic Load/serving	16
Calories	210 Cal
Total Fat	2.7 g
Cholesterol	0mg
Sodium	8 mg
Total Carbohydrates	41 g
Dietary fibers	1.8g
Sugars	1.7 g
Protein	4.5 g
Vitamin C	14%
Vitamin A	3%
Iron	5%
Calcium	3%

Ingredients

- 2 cups basmati rice
- 4 cups water
- 1 teaspoon cumin seeds
- 4 teaspoon oil
- 1 onion chopped
- 1 cup frozen green peas
- 1 bay leaf
- Salt and Pepper to taste
- 1/2 teaspoon lemon juice

Method

- Wash and Soak the rice 1/2 hour prior to cooking.
- Heat oil in a pan and sauté the onions to little brown.
- Add water and lemon juice then bring it to a boil.
- Add the green peas and rice and boil for 3 minutes.
- Drain the upper water with the help of a colander.
- Add 1 cup of water and bring to a boil.
- Cover the pan and allow the rice to cook for 4 minutes.
- Heat oil in a small pan and splutter cumin seeds.
- Sprinkle on the rice.
- Serve hot with gravy.

TIP: The lemon juice is added to prevent the rice from sticking and the water is drained to remove starch.

19. Kidney Beans

Preparation time	10 minutes
Ready time	30 minutes
Serves	4
Serving quantity/unit	200 G/7.1oz
Glycemic index/serving	19±2
Glycemic Load/serving	7
Calories	250 Cal
Total Fat	7.6 g
Cholesterol	0mg
Sodium	16 mg
Total Carbohydrates	36.5 g
Dietary fibers	8.8g
Sugars	5.0 g
Protein	11.1 g
Vitamin C	24%
Vitamin A	10%
Iron	21%
Calcium	6%

Ingredients

- 1 cup kidney beans

- 2 onion
- 2 tablespoon oil
- 1 teaspoon ginger paste
- 1 teaspoon garlic paste
- 1 teaspoon cumin seeds
- Salt and Pepper to taste
- 2 tomatoes diced
- 1 bay leaf
- Coriander leaves

Method

- Soak the kidney beans overnight for best results.
- Heat oil in a saucepan and sauté the onions till brown.
- Add the ginger and garlic and stir.
- Add tomatoes, salt, pepper and bay leaf and keep on stirring till the oil is separated.
- Add 2 cups water along with the kidney beans and simmer.
- Reduce the heat and simmer the kidney beans 40 minutes.
- Dry extra water till the gravy thickens.
- Serve hot after garnishing with coriander.

TIP: If you forget to soak the kidney beans add 1/2 teaspoon of soda bicarbonate to make the kidney beans tender.

Dinner

20. Penne with Vegetables

Preparation time	15 minutes
Ready time	30 minutes
Serves	4
Serving quantity/unit	300 G/10.6oz
Glycemic index/serving	39±4
Glycemic Load/serving	17
Calories	216 Cal
Total Fat	2.0 g
Cholesterol	41mg
Sodium	62 mg
Total Carbohydrates	39.4 g
Dietary fibers	1.7g
Sugars	2.3 g
Protein	9.1 g
Vitamin C	99%
Vitamin A	22%
Iron	14%
Calcium	3%

Ingredients

- 1 cup broccoli, cut in florets
- 2 teaspoon garlic
- Oregano 1 tablespoon
- Red pepper 1/2 teaspoon
- 2 cups mushrooms, chopped
- 2 tablespoon dry white wine
- 2 tablespoon chopped olives
- 2 Tomatoes chopped
- 8 ounce penne, boiled and drained
- Salt and Pepper to taste
- 1 teaspoon lemon juice

Method

- Boil broccoli, drain and keep aside.

- Heat oil in a pan and olive oil.
- Add garlic, oregano, lemon juice and red pepper.
- Add mushrooms and stir and cover and simmer for 2 minutes.
- Add wine and simmer for 2 minutes.
- Add broccoli, olives and tomatoes.
- Take a large bowl and mix the penne with the vegetables, lemon juice and olive oil and toss well. Serve warm.

TIP: Vegetables provide complete nutrition so this dish is an asset for people who want to lose weight.

21. Chili Beef Noodles

Preparation time	10 minutes
Ready time	25 minutes
Serves	4
Serving quantity/unit	300 G/10.6oz
Glycemic index/serving	42±4
Glycemic Load/serving	19
Calories	450 Cal
Total Fat	8.1 g
Cholesterol	59mg
Sodium	606 mg
Total Carbohydrates	43.4 g
Dietary fibers	2.6g
Sugars	1.7 g
Protein	28.1 g
Vitamin C	5%
Vitamin A	3%
Iron	29%
Calcium	4%

Ingredients

- 1 sirloin steak, trimmed
- 1/2 cup spring onion chopped
- 1 tablespoon oil
- 2 capsicum julienned
- 2 red chilies
- Salt and Pepper to taste
- 1 teaspoon lemon juice

- 2 cups vegetable stock
- 1 teaspoon ginger shredded
- 2 teaspoon soya sauce
- 300 g thin noodles

Method

- Boil the spring onions along with the stock, ginger and chilies.
- Cook the steak on a pan till medium rare.
- Add the noodles to the stock and cook for around 3 minutes.
- Add salt and pepper and mix till a little.
- Add the noodles in a serving bowl and top it with the steak slices with capsicum.
- Garnish with soya sauce and serve.

TIP: The beef can be replaced with chicken or mutton steaks.

22. Cumberland Fish Pie

Preparation time	5 minutes
Ready time	10 minutes
Serves	20 portions
Serving quantity/unit	100 G/3.5oz
Glycemic index/serving	59±4
Glycemic Load/serving	14
Calories	90 Cal
Total Fat	3.7 g
Cholesterol	8mg
Sodium	56 mg
Total Carbohydrates	12.4 g
Dietary fibers	1.3g
Sugars	0.5 g
Protein	3.1 g
Vitamin C	17%
Vitamin A	0%
Iron	3%
Calcium	1%

Ingredients

- 2 tablespoons oil
- 1 onion, finely chopped
- 250 g fish fillet(minced)

- 1 tablespoon all purpose flour
- 2 cups of vegetable stock
- 1 kg potato
- 1 tablespoon butter

Method

- Preheat the oven to 180 degrees.
- In a pan sauté the onions until brown and then add the fish and cook for a while.
- Add the flour and stir fry.
- Add the stock and allow it to simmer for around 10 minutes.
- Cook the potatoes in boiling water till they are tender.
- Peel the potatoes and mash them.
- Take a pie dish and add the fish mixture in it.
- Top the fish with a layer of mashed potatoes and bake.
- Bake for 30 minutes till the top layer becomes brownish.
- Serve hot.

TIP: Fish is a low source of carbohydrates and rich in proteins. A mixture of Vegetables can replace the fish for a vegan diet of low glycemic load.

23. Vegetable Burger

Preparation time	5 minutes
Ready time	10 minutes
Serves	4
Serving quantity/unit	100 G/3.5oz
Glycemic index/serving	59±4
Glycemic Load/serving	14
Calories	270 Cal
Total Fat	9.7 g
Cholesterol	42mg
Sodium	262 mg
Total Carbohydrates	40.4 g
Dietary fibers	3.3g
Sugars	5.5 g
Protein	6.1 g
Vitamin C	31%
Vitamin A	106%
Iron	11%
Calcium	5%

Ingredients

For the Pattie

- 2 cups grated potatoes
- 2 carrots grated
- 1 teaspoon ginger garlic paste
- 1 egg
- 3 tablespoon all purpose flour
- Oil to fry

For the Burger

- Vegetable Pattie (As made above)
- Lettuce leaves
- 1 tomato(sliced)
- Sweet chili sauce
- 4 Burger buns

Method

For the Pattie

- Mix all the ingredients in the list of Pattie and shape the mid into round burger patties.
- Fry the Patties in minimal oil.
- Drain on paper towels.

For the Burger

- Take a Burger bun and slit it.
- Keep the burger Pattie on one side.
- Top it up with lettuce leaves, tomatoes and chili sauce.
- Enjoy your burger.

TIP: The Patties mixture should not be too moist and not too hard. If it is too hard add some water and if too moist add little bread crumbs.

24. Hamburger

Preparation time	5 minutes
Ready time	10 minutes
Serves	4
Serving quantity/unit	100 G/3.5oz
Glycemic index/serving	59±4
Glycemic Load/serving	14
Calories	320 Cal
Total Fat	17.3 g
Cholesterol	190mg
Sodium	216 mg
Total Carbohydrates	14.4 g
Dietary fibers	1.4g
Sugars	3.5 g
Protein	42.1 g
Vitamin C	10%
Vitamin A	56%
Iron	30%
Calcium	5%

Ingredients

For the Pattie

- 500 G beef
- 1 onion
- 1 stock cube
- 2 tablespoon tomato sauce
- 2 teaspoon garlic paste
- 2 tablespoon all purpose flour
- 2 eggs
- 1 teaspoon coriander
- 1 carrot finely grated
- Oil to fry

For the Burger

- Beef Pattie (As made above)
- Lettuce leaves
- 1 tomato(sliced)

- Sweet chili sauce
- Burger buns

Method

For the Pattie

- Mix all the ingredients in the list of Pattie and shape the mid into round hamburger patties.
- Fry the Patties in minimal oil.
- Drain on paper towels.
- Wash the vegetables and chop them roughly.
- Add them in a blender along with the lemon and ginger juice.
- Add salt and pepper and mix till a smooth blend is formed.
- Serve chilled with ice cubes.

For the Burger

- Take a Burger bun and slit it.
- Keep the burger Pattie on one side.
- Top it up with lettuce leaves, tomatoes and chili sauce.
- Enjoy your burger.

TIP: Burger with cheese and mayonnaise generally is high in glycemic load so they should be avoided…

25. Beef and ale Casserole

Preparation time	20 minutes
Ready time	180 minutes
Serves	8
Serving quantity/unit	300 G/10.6oz
Glycemic index/serving	53±4
Glycemic Load/serving	8
Calories	305 Cal
Total Fat	9.4 g
Cholesterol	100mg
Sodium	122 mg
Total Carbohydrates	12.6 g
Dietary fibers	2.3g
Sugars	5.5 g
Protein	36.1 g
Vitamin C	32%
Vitamin A	59%
Iron	23%
Calcium	5%

Ingredients

- 900g beef steak
- 4 teaspoon oil
- 2 onions chopped
- 3 turnips peeled and cut into halves
- 1 cup chopped mushrooms
- 2 carrots chopped
- 600 ml ale
- 3 tomatoes, chopped
- 1 teaspoon honey
- 2 bay leaves
- Salt and Pepper to taste
- 1 teaspoon lemon juice

Method

- Heat oil in a pan and cook the beef to a golden brown.
- Lay the beef in a casserole dish.
- In the pan now sauté the onions and turnips and then add mushrooms and cook for 3 minutes, and then add in the casserole.

- Now lay the carrots along with the ale, tomatoes honey and bay leaf in the casserole.
- Cover and cook in the oven for about 2 hours or till the meat are tender.
- Serve the stew with bread or squeak cakes.

TIP: The whole-meal barley bread has a low Glycemic Load of '5' and goes well with this recipe. White bread has a higher Glycemic Load.

26. Tomato and herb chicken

Preparation time	20 minutes
Ready time	80 minutes
Serves	4
Serving quantity/unit	250 G/8.8oz
Glycemic index/serving	29±4
Glycemic Load/serving	9
Calories	200 Cal
Total Fat	7.7 g
Cholesterol	48mg
Sodium	66 mg
Total Carbohydrates	8.8 g
Dietary fibers	1.8g
Sugars	3.3 g
Protein	24.7 g
Vitamin C	2%
Vitamin A	27%
Iron	8%
Calcium	2%

Ingredients

- 2 garlic cloves
- 1/2 teaspoon oregano
- 1/2 teaspoon paprika
- 2 tablespoon oil
- 2 tablespoon all purpose flour
- 2 boneless skinless breasts
- 4 tomatoes, diced
- 1 tablespoon parsley
- Salt and Pepper to taste

Method

- Mix the butter garlic, oregano, paprika in a bowl. Add salt and pepper.
- Heat the oven to 80 degrees.
- Coat the chicken pieces evenly with all purpose flour.
- In a pan heat oil and fry the chicken pieces so as to make them brown on both sides.
- Keep the chicken in an oven-proof tray and let the pieces be warm.
- In the pan heat the butter and oregano and add tomatoes and let them fry till they become tender.
- Allow the sauce to thicken and then pour on the chicken breasts and serve.
- Garnish with parsley leaves and serve hot.

TIP: The chicken breasts should be softened with a mallet if required prior to use.

Deserts

27. Apple Berry Crumble

Preparation time	15 minutes
Ready time	70 minutes
Serves	8
Serving quantity/unit	150 G/5.3oz
Glycemic index/serving	41±3
Glycemic Load/serving	14
Calories	176 Cal
Total Fat	3.4 g
Cholesterol	8mg
Sodium	22 mg
Total Carbohydrates	22.7 g
Dietary fibers	2.6g
Sugars	14g
Protein	1.1g
Vitamin C	17%
Vitamin A	3%
Iron	3%
Calcium	1%

Ingredients

- 1/2 cup apple juice
- 3 apples sliced

- 1/2 cup chopped pear
- 2 tablespoons honey
- 1/3 cup oats
- 4 tablespoons of wheat flour
- 1 teaspoon cinnamon
- Pinch of nutmeg
- 2 tablespoon butter

Method

- Combine the apple juice with the dried strawberries in a bowl.
- In a baking dish arrange the sliced apple and sprinkle them with honey.
- Pour the apple juice mix on these pears.
- Mix the oats with the wheat flour and nutmeg and cinnamon.
- Add butter to this mixture and sprinkle over the apples.
- Bake the dish in an oven at 350 degree for around 30 to 40 minutes or until the surface of the crumble is brown.
- Serve warm.

TIP: The apples in this crumble can be replaced by pears too.

28. Mixed Berry Mousse

Preparation time	10 minutes
Ready time	20 minutes
Serves	8
Serving quantity/unit	50G/1.8oz
Glycemic index/serving	36±3
Glycemic Load/serving	4
Calories	43 Cal
Total Fat	0.2 g
Cholesterol	0mg
Sodium	28 mg
Total Carbohydrates	8.8 g
Dietary fibers	1.9g
Sugars	6.1g
Protein	2.2g
Vitamin C	20%
Vitamin A	1%
Iron	2%
Calcium	1%

Ingredients

- 3 cups of mixed berries, chopped
- 3 teaspoon honey
- 4 egg whites
- 1 tablespoon lemon juice

Method

- Boil the mixed berries in a pan of water.
- Simmer and cook till the berries are tender.
- Turn off the heat when the berries become soft and drain them.
- Do not throw the left over liquid.
- Separate the egg whites and add fresh lemon juice to them and whisk in a blender.
- Add sugar to this and whisk the whole mixture spoon by spoon so as to form a perfect blend.
- Spoon the mixture in tall glasses and serve by adding juice and fresh berries.

TIP: Chocolate mousse is also made in the same way.

29. Doughnut

Preparation time	20 minutes
Ready time	30 minutes
Serves	12
Serving quantity/unit	50G/1.8oz
Glycemic index/serving	75±7
Glycemic Load/serving	15
Calories	156 Cal
Total Fat	5.0 g
Cholesterol	20 mg
Sodium	36mg
Total Carbohydrates	25 g
Dietary fibers	0.6g
Sugars	9g
Protein	3.2g
Vitamin C	0%
Vitamin A	2%
Iron	6%
Calcium	7%

Ingredients

- 2 cups All-purpose flour
- 1 tablespoon baking powder
- 1/2 cup sugar
- Pinch of Salt
- 1/4 teaspoon cardamom powder
- 2 tablespoons of butter
- 1/2 cup milk
- 1 egg
- Oil for frying

Method

- Mix sugar, flour, baking powder, salt along with cardamom powder.
- Add butter to this mixture.
- Add milk and eggs and mix well.
- Knead the dough softly.
- Make rolls of about 1 cm thickness and cut a hole in it.
- Heat the oil in a fryer and fry the doughnuts till golden brown.
- Drain and Serve.

TIP: Sugar and chocolate coated donuts amount to a higher GI Load hence should be avoided.

30. Low-Fat Vanilla Custard

Preparation time	30 minutes
Ready time	240 minutes
Serves	4
Serving quantity/unit	220mL/7.5 fl oz
Glycemic index/serving	45±3
Glycemic Load/serving	11
Calories	186 Cal
Total Fat	7.8 g
Cholesterol	150 mg
Sodium	157mg
Total Carbohydrates	19.8 g
Dietary fibers	0g
Sugars	14.2g
Protein	11.8g
Vitamin C	0%
Vitamin A	13%
Iron	5%
Calcium	24%

Ingredients

- 3 teaspoon honey
- 3 tablespoons cornstarch
- 4 egg yolks
- 1/2 Liter(3 cups) low fat milk
- 2 teaspoon butter
- 2 teaspoons vanilla essence

Method

- Boil milk along with cornstarch, yolks, salt and honey in a pan with a heavy bottom.
- Stir till the liquid thickens for about 25 minutes.
- Remove from heat and let the mixture stand after adding butter and Vanilla essence.
- Cover the custard and keep it for 2 hours to chill.
- Garnish with chopped almonds or cinnamon powder.
- Serve chilled.

TIP: Vanilla essence can be replaced by rose essence. Fresh fruits can be incorporated in the custard except banana and mango as they tend to increase the Glycemic load.

31. Rice Pudding Caramel

Preparation time	30 minutes
Ready time	240 minutes
Serves	4
Serving quantity/unit	189G/6.7oz
Glycemic index/serving	41±3
Glycemic Load/serving	16
Calories	222 Cal
Total Fat	8.2 g
Cholesterol	16 mg
Sodium	100 mg
Total Carbohydrates	39.1g
Dietary fibers	0g
Sugars	26.3 g
Protein	6.2g
Vitamin C	0%
Vitamin A	5%
Iron	3%
Calcium	17%

Ingredients

- 500 ml milk(low fat)
- 1/3 cup of broken rice
- Pinch of salt
- 1/4 cup sugar
- 1/2 cup caramel ice cream
- 1/4 teaspoon cardamom powder
- 2 teaspoon raisins

Method

- Boil milk along with rice, cardamom and salt in a heavy bottomed saucepan.
- Reduce the heat and simmer for about 25 minutes.
- Keep on stirring the pudding to prevent the rice from sticking to the bottom.
- When the rice becomes tender remove the pan from the heat.
- Mix the caramel ice cream and raisins with the pudding and keep aside.
- Add the sugar to a thick bottomed pan and heat at medium till brown.
- Reduce heat and stir till sugar melts and pour on the pudding.
- Refrigerate the pudding and serve chilled.

TIP: Puddings can be made from the readymade packets available but the contents should be taken into account.

32. Rice Pudding cinnamon flavored

Preparation time	30 minutes
Ready time	240 minutes
Serves	4
Serving quantity/unit	160mL/5.4 fl oz
Glycemic index/serving	52±4
Glycemic Load/serving	19
Calories	138 Cal
Total Fat	2.6 g
Cholesterol	10 mg
Sodium	93 mg
Total Carbohydrates	32.0 g
Dietary fibers	0g
Sugars	19.9 g
Protein	5.2g
Vitamin C	0%
Vitamin A	5%
Iron	4%
Calcium	16%

Ingredients

- 500 ml milk(low fat)
- 1/3 cup of broken rice
- Pinch of salt
- 1/4 cup sugar
- 1/2 teaspoon cinnamon powder
- 2 teaspoon raisins

Method

- Boil milk along with rice and salt in a heavy bottomed saucepan.
- Reduce the heat and simmer for about 25 minutes.
- Keep on stirring the pudding to prevent the rice from sticking to the bottom.
- When the rice becomes tender remove the pan from the heat.
- Add the sugar, raisins and cinnamon and mix properly.
- Heat the pan again and let the pudding thicken.

- Refrigerate the pudding and serve chilled.

TIP: Fruits like mango and banana should not be added in the pudding as they may increase the Glycemic Load of the pudding.

33. Chocolate Butterscotch Muffin

Preparation time	15 minutes
Ready time	35 minutes
Serves	12
Serving quantity/unit	59G/2.1oz
Glycemic index/serving	53±5
Glycemic Load/serving	15
Calories	196 Cal
Total Fat	7.3 g
Cholesterol	49mg
Sodium	363 mg
Total Carbohydrates	40 g
Dietary fibers	1.6g
Sugars	22g
Protein	4.9g
Vitamin C	0%
Vitamin A	3%
Iron	11%
Calcium	1%

Ingredients

- 2 cups all purpose flour
- 1/2 cup cocoa powder
- 1 cup sugar
- 1 tablespoon baking soda
- Pinch of salt
- 3 tablespoon butter
- 3 eggs
- 1 cup butterscotch and chocolate chips
- 2 teaspoons vanilla essence

Method

- Preheat the oven to 425 degrees.

- Mix all the dry ingredients in a bowl.
- Mix the wet ingredients and add to the dry ingredients to form a uniform mixture.
- Now add the chocolate and butterscotch chips and stir evenly and slowly.
- Divide the batter evenly in 12 muffins in the baking tray.
- Bake the muffins for around 18 to 20 minutes till done.

TIP: The chocolate chips can be substituted with chopped nuts in order to get nutty muffins.

Exclusive Bonus Download: Gluten Free Living Secrets

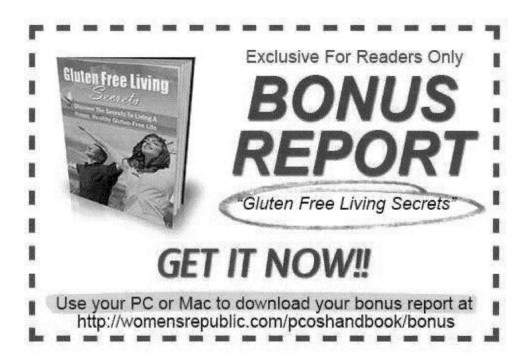

Download your bonus, please visit the download link above from your PC or MAC. To open PDF files, visit http://get.adobe.com/reader/ to download the reader if it's not already installed on your PC or Mac. To open ZIP files, you may need to download WinZip from http://www.winzip.com. This download is for PC or Mac ONLY and might not be downloadable to kindle.

Are you sick and tired of trying every weight loss program out there and failing to see results? Or are you frustrated with not feeling as energetic as you used to despite what you eat? Perhaps you always seem to have a bit of a " dodgy stomach " and indigestion seems to be a regular part of your life?

There's nothing worse than sitting down to a nice big plate of pasta and enjoying your meal only to be met with a growling stomach and the inevitable rush to the toilet.

It's that bloated feeling you get after eating a piece of bread that just " doesn't seem right " . Almost as if you've eaten something poisonous.

Gluten Free Living Secrets is a complete resource that will tell you everything you need to know about the dangers of eating gluten and how to go about transitioning yourself and your family to a life free of this dangerous substance.

Here's just a taste of what you will discover inside Gluten Free Living Secrets:

- What foods you should focus on when first switching to a gluten-free diet
- The 9 grains that are safe and gluten-free
- The truth about whether you can eat pasta on a gluten-free diet
- What you should know to determine if you have Celiac Disease
- and that's not all...
- Why you may want to consider eliminating gluten from your child's diet
- The top 10 reasons to go gluten-free
- How to transform your pantry to be gluten-free
- A list of essential gluten-free shopping tips
- How to keep your kids happy around their gluten-eating friends
- Tips on staying gluten-free when eating out

Gluten Free Living Secrets comes in a digital PDF format that is easy to read either on your computer or on your eBook reader.

Visit the URL above to download this guide and start achieving your overall health and weight loss goals NOW

One Last Thing...

Thank you so much for reading my book. I hope you really liked it. As you probably know, many people look at the reviews on Amazon before they decide to purchase a book. If you liked the book, could you please take a minute to leave a review with your feedback? 60 seconds is all I'm asking for, and it would mean the world to me.

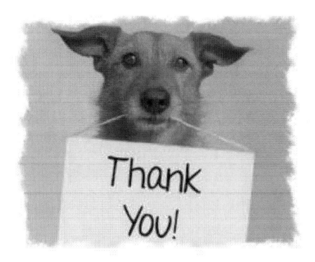

✶✶✶✶✶✶

Closing Author's Note

I hope you have enjoyed reading this book and that it has motivated you take the necessary steps towards a healthier, happier you. As I mentioned at the beginning of the book, if you haven't already read my first book on PCOS "*Permanently Beat PCOS: The Complete Solution*" and are still keen to gain a more in-depth understanding of the condition and other methods, supplements and lifestyle changes you should be making then pick up your copy from your favorite online marketplace now.

Books by This Author:

Permanently Beat Bacterial Vaginosis

Permanently Beat Yeast Infection & Candida

Permanently Beat Urinary Tract Infections

Permanently Beat Hypothyroidism Naturally

Permanently Beat PCOS

The Permanently Beat PCOS Diet & Exercise Shortcuts

About the Author

Caroline D. Greene is a mother of 2 wonderful girls and a wife to a supportive husband. She has dedicated the past seven years to researching the various women's health topics that are not being openly discussed and providing help and support to the women dealing with these issues in their daily life.

Caroline D. Greene

Published by Women's Republic

Atlanta, Georgia USA

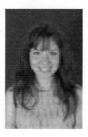

Copyright © 2012 Caroline D. Greene

Images and Cover by Women's Republic

Made in the USA
Lexington, KY
15 July 2013